Ventilator Modes Made Easy

An Easy to Understand Guide to a Topic That Is Never Well Explained

By Damon Wiseley B.H.S.c., RRT

http://www.respiratythera
pyprograms.com

I0391053

The reader is responsible for his or her own actions.

Adherence to all applicable laws and regulations, including international, federal, state, and local governing professional licensing, business practices, advertising, and all other aspects of doing business and providing care to patients in the US, Canada, or any other jurisdiction is the sole responsibility of the purchaser or reader.

Neither the author nor the publisher assumes any responsibility or liability whatsoever on the behalf of the purchaser or reader of these materials. The medical information provided in this book is, at best, of a general nature and cannot substitute for the advice of a medical professional. Although the author has made every effort to ensure that the information in this book was correct at press time, the author does not assume and hereby disclaim any liability to any party for any loss, damage, or disruption caused by errors or

Table of Contents

Introduction

About This Book

Congratulations on purchasing this book and beginning your journey to a better understanding of ventilator modes! The work you do is vitally important to your patients' health and happiness, and I commend you on striving to be the best you can be!

Let's face it; ventilators can be confusing and even scary to deal with. It seems every year, there is a new mode or hybrid mode introduced, a new weaning parameter to measure, or a new buzzword to wrap your head around.

This book reviews, in simple language the basic knowledge to understand ventilator settings. Ventilator settings made easy includes the mechanical settings you input and patient data you must measure and interpret. This book will provide you with a sound understanding of conventional modes of ventilation and advanced modes. My goal is for you to learn and retain this information, rather than trying to memorize it.

In all honesty, some material in this book will demand your attention and may seem intimidating at first. That is just the brutal reality we face when trying to learn something hard. However, my goal is to break down all this information into simple language.

As always, follow your hospital's protocols and the direction of a qualified physician when using any mode of ventilation in this book.

About Me

I'm a Registered Respiratory Therapist. Over the past fifteen years, I have worked alongside some of the best nurses, doctors, and respiratory therapists in many critical care settings, including the ICU, E.R., and even Neonatal Transport teams. One thing I have noticed, working with these professionals, is that many wish they had a better understanding of ventilator modes. Because ventilator modes are one of the most important things to understand when using mechanical ventilation, I felt it would be helpful to provide a review of the most common modes you will encounter.

Ventilator Basics

When choosing a ventilator mode, you are choosing how a patient's breathing will be supported. Making the right choice starts with two basic questions. Do you want the patient to be completely supported by the machine, or can they do some of the breathing on their own? Should you control the pressure or the volume inside the lungs?

Aside from these two basic questions, mode selection then typically becomes based on the clinician's familiarity with the mode and the hospital's particular preferences. There is a high amount of variation in the modes used throughout the world. Therefore, understanding how each mode works, how to select each mode's settings, and when to use each mode is important to both your career and your patient's health.

However, before we dive into these topics, there are several fundamental concepts and terms that, if fully understood, will help you along the way.

First, when we place our patients on mechanical ventilation, we are trying to control their ventilation and oxygenation.

1. **Ventilation** controls the carbon dioxide level (PCO2) and is equal to the volume of air you move in and out of the lungs. More air in and out = more ventilation = getting rid of more PCO2.

2. **Oxygenation** is controlled by the FiO2 and PEEP settings. Oxygen diffuses into the lungs through the alveolar capillary membrane.

Second, ventilator modes are then classified as:

1. **Volume Control Modes** - This category of modes gives a set volume with each machine-delivered breath. With volume-limited modes, the volume is set

and remains constant, while the pressure inside the lungs will vary.

2. **Pressure Control Modes** - This category of modes gives a set pressure with each machine-delivered breath. With pressure-limited modes, the pressure is set and remains constant, while the volume delivered with each breath will vary.

3. **Dual Control Modes** - These combine the characteristics of both volume and pressure control modes.

<u>**Finally**</u>, before we review the modes, here is some basic terminology you should familiarize yourself with:

Tidal volume - This is simply the size of the breath as measured in milliliters. Tidal volume is often calculated based on a patient's ideal body weight. Different lung pathologies will require different sized tidal volumes. Patients with stiff lungs, such as those with ARDS, are treated with tidal volumes lower than those with healthy lungs.

Respiratory rate or frequency - This is a measure of how many breaths a patient takes per minute. Rate can be expressed as either the set rate or the total rate. The set rate represents the minimum breaths the ventilator will give per minute. The total rate is equal to the set rate, plus whatever additional breaths the patient takes within that minute.

Minute volume - Rate x tidal volume = minute volume. This is the amount of air you move in and out of the patient's lungs each minute.

PEEP (positive end expiratory pressure) - PEEP is the amount of pressure left inside the lungs after the patient has fully exhaled. To help you understand PEEP, picture that point when you begin to blow up a balloon. Picture what the balloon looks like when it goes from hanging from your mouth to sticking straight out just before it expands. That is a good representation of what PEEP is and what it does to alveoli. PEEP helps keep the alveoli patent and prevents them from collapsing. PEEP can also recruit alveoli by opening them up after they have collapsed.

A PEEP level of 2 – 3 cm H20 pressure is naturally present in all of us. However, when an advanced airway, such as an endotracheal tube, is placed our naturally occurring PEEP is lost. The only way to get it back is to add PEEP from a mechanical ventilator.

Trigger - The trigger is whatever makes the ventilator give a breath. You can choose between a flow, pressure, or time trigger. A flow trigger occurs when the machine senses the patient initiating a breath by detecting a change in flow within the ventilator circuit. A pressure trigger occurs when the machine senses a change in pressure within the ventilator circuit. A time trigger occurs simply when the patient is due for another breath based on the respiratory rate and other settings you have picked.

Cycle - Cycling refers to what makes the ventilator stop giving the breath. Cycling ends the machine-delivered breath and allows the patient to exhale.

Volume Control Modes

Assist Control Mode (A/C)

Assist control is the most popular mode of ventilation used in critical care. This is because A/C mode gives near maximal ventilatory support to the patient. In A/C mode, the patient receives the full set tidal volume for each machine set breath *and* for each spontaneous breath they take. Patients on A/C mode may breathe as much as they desire, and when they do, the machine will support them entirely. Assist control mode is often referred to as continuous mandatory ventilation (CMV) or volume control (VC).

When is A/C mode used? A/C mode is often used when full ventilator support is desired. Because A/C mode provides a preset tidal volume with both the machine set breaths and the patients spontaneous breaths, it imposes the least work on the patient. This makes it an excellent initial mode for a most patients.

Important notes regarding A/C mode: Some patients on A/C mode might breathe too fast above the respiratory rate you have set. This may cause them to hyperventilate. Patients with end-stage liver disease, head trauma, or in the hyper-ventilatory stage of sepsis may do this. Also, when using A/C mode, you must always remember the pressure inside the patient's lungs can quickly change. This is because in A/C mode, the ventilator does not care about the pressure inside the patient's lungs. The ventilator only cares about the volume when in A/C mode. Because of this, the high peak airway pressure limit must be set to a suitable level to avoid delivering excessive pressure to the patient's lungs.

How does A/C mode work?

The ventilator will deliver a breath in A/C mode whenever there is a patient trigger or a time trigger. The patient triggered breaths account for the assist part of assist control. The time triggered breaths account for the control part of assist control. A patient trigger occurs when the ventilator senses a patient's effort to breathe. The ventilator senses the patient's effort by reading a change in the pressure or flow within the ventilator circuit. The flow trigger or pressure trigger is often set by the respiratory therapist, as is the sensitivity of each trigger. A time trigger occurs when the patient is due for a breath, based on the respiratory rate set. For example, if you set the respiratory rate at 20 breaths per minute, the ventilator will give a time-triggered breath every three seconds.

Regardless of how the breath is triggered, as soon as it is triggered, the ventilator will take over for the patient and deliver a full set tidal volume by applying a constant rate of flow. When the preset tidal volume is delivered, flow will stop and the patient can exhale passively. Assist control mode is a patient or time-triggered, constant flow, volume-cycled mode of ventilation.

SIMV Mode

Synchronized intermittent mandatory ventilation is a long name for a fairly simple mode. In SIMV, the patient gets full tidal volume support for the set breaths, while additional breaths the patient takes are unsupported. The machine will do nothing for the patient when they take a spontaneous breath above the respiratory rate you have set. The volume of the breath the patient gets will only be what they can generate. This creates more work for the patient as compared to assist control mode. This increased workload may be good for the patient or bad, depending on their condition.

One thing we can do in SIMV mode to support the patient's spontaneous breaths and reduce their work of breathing is to add pressure support ventilation or PSV. PSV is covered in detail later in this book. Also, some ventilators have combined the synchronization and spontaneous breathing capabilities of SIMV with pressure control ventilation.

When is SIMV used? Because SIMV causes an increased work of breathing at lower set rates and may lead to muscle fatigue, it is not normally selected as the initial mode of ventilation. Instead, SIMV has been commonly used late in a patient's ICU course. Some clinicians and hospitals use it to recondition pulmonary musculature and to wean patients from the ventilator. However, this approach is controversial, as studies have shown this prolongs the time to extubation. SIMV as a mode for weaning is now considered outdated. Some physicians have found SIMV to be useful when used for patients who hyperventilate on assist control mode.

How does SIMV mode work? The most important thing to know about SIMV is that the spontaneous breaths are not supported by the machine, unless pressure support is added. Understanding exactly how SIMV synchronizes its breaths is actually fairly complicated.

I know many smart doctors and respiratory therapists who still have trouble accurately explaining how SIMV works. However, for those of you who really want to understand this, keep reading.

Despite the title of this book, there really is no easy way to explain how the SIMV mode works. To understand exactly how SIMV works, you have to understand first what a breath cycle and interval time is. A complete breath cycle is equal to 60 seconds divided by the set respiratory rate. So if a patient had a set respiratory rate of 12 breaths per minute, the breath cycle time would be 5 seconds because $60 \div 12 = 5$ seconds. In SIMV, the breath cycle is then divided into the mandatory interval and the spontaneous interval. *If the patient initiates a spontaneous breath during the mandatory interval, they will get*

a full set tidal volume. If the patient initiates a spontaneous breath during the spontaneous interval, then they will get no support. The spontaneous breaths taken during the spontaneous interval of the breath cycle are not supported. The only machine support they will receive when taking a spontaneous breath during the spontaneous interval of the breath cycle is if pressure support is added to the vent settings.

Pressure Control Modes

Pressure Control (PC)

In pressure control mode, the ventilator delivers a set pressure, instead of a set tidal volume. The pressure delivered to the patient's lungs remains the same with each breath. This is what makes pressure control an attractive mode to use, particularly in patients with stiff lungs. However, as we gain control of the pressure, we lose control of the volume. The volume will vary, depending on the compliance and resistance in the patient's lungs and within the ventilator circuit. Therefore, monitoring the volumes in your patient is vitally important, as many things can cause changes in compliance and resistance (a kinked ETT tube, bronchospasm, secretions in the airways, mucous plugs, pneumothorax, ARDS etc.)

All these things can cause a very sudden and serious drop in your patient's ventilation.

When is PC mode used? Limiting the pressures applied inside the lungs results in less risk for pressure related lung injury such as barotrauma or damage to the alveoli. Therefore, pressure control mode is often used in patients in whom the pressure inside the lungs must be controlled, such as ARDS.

How do you set up pressure control? Most clinicians are unsure exactly how to set the inspiratory pressure level when first using pressure control. A common starting point is to set the inspiratory pressure at 20 cm H20 and titrate that pressure to achieve the volumes appropriate for the patient. This is more a rule of thumb type approach rather than a scientifically proven approach. Another method of choosing the initial inspiratory pressure setting is to set it 3 - 5 cm H20 pressure above the mean airway pressure and then titrate the pressure up or down as needed.

Important notes: I cannot stress enough that you must always be aware that the volume is variable in pressure control mode. Setting your alarm limits appropriately for both tidal volume and minute ventilation is vital to avoid hypo-ventilating your patient.

How exactly does PC mode work? An inspiratory pressure is set instead of a tidal volume. When a breath is patient or time-triggered, pressure is maintained at a constant level with a decelerating flow rate. The breath is delivered until the upper pressure limit is exceeded or the preset I-time is reached. At this point, the ventilator cycles the breath off, and exhalation begins

APRV Mode

Airway pressure release ventilation allows spontaneous breathing, while alternating between a high and a low pressure. The high pressure is held for a long time and then released to a lower pressure for a short time. The release time is so short it prevents complete emptying of the lungs and intentionally causes auto-PEEP. This normally would be very uncomfortable for the patient. However, because they may breathe spontaneously at any point in the breath cycle, this mode is generally tolerated. The spontaneous breaths can be supported with the addition of pressure support. The total respiratory rate is not set directly and is a product of the set inspiratory and expiratory times.

When is APRV mode used? APRV mode is often used as a rescue mode in patients with acute respiratory distress syndrome (ARDS) who are difficult to oxygenate. Though some small studies have consistently shown an improvement in oxygenation and a lower requirement for sedatives, none have shown evidence of reduced mortality when using this mode. APRV has not been studied in patients with COPD or neuromuscular disease and is not appropriate in patients requiring deep sedation.

Important notes regarding APRV: Different manufacturers have created modes similar to APRV. These modes include: BiLevel (Covidien), APRV (Dräger), Bi-Vent (Maquet), BiPhasic (CareFusion), and DuoPAP (Hamilton).

How does APRV work? APRV uses long inflation periods and high mean airway pressures to achieve alveolar recruitment. APRV delivers time-triggered, pressure-controlled, time-cycled mandatory set breaths, while allowing the patient to breathe spontaneously at any point in the ventilatory cycle.

No consensus exists regarding the initial setup and application of APRV. Therefore, initial settings and ventilation strategies are largely determined by clinician familiarity and hospital preference. With that said, here are some general guidelines recommended by some authors regarding the parameters that must be chosen. As always, follow your hospital's protocols and the direction of a qualified physician when using this or any other mode of ventilation in this book.

Regardless of the ventilator brand used, four general settings applied in APRV.

1. Inflation pressure or P-high - The inflation pressure (P-high) is set to deliver an inflation pressure of 4-8 ml's per kilo of the patient's body weight, while limiting total applied pressure to less than 35cm H20. The inflation time is set to allow the longest inflation time while still achieving the desired minute ventilation.

2. Deflation pressure or P-low -
    The deflation pressure (P-low)
    is set between 0 and 8 cm-H20.
    P-low is PEEP.

3. Inflation time or T-high - The
    inflation time (T-high) is set to
    allow the longest inflation time
    while still achieving the desired
    minute ventilation.

4. Deflation time or T-low -
    Deflation time (T-low) is set
    from 0.5 to 1 second.

SIMV-PC Mode

Some ventilator manufacturers
have combined the
synchronization and spontaneous
breathing characteristics unique to
SIMV with pressure control
ventilation. In this mode,
spontaneous breathing can be
supported with pressure support,
just like in SIMV. However, like
pressure control mode, an
inspiratory pressure, rather than a
tidal volume, is set.

Dual Control Modes

Dual control modes use computer algorithms to deliver the best of both worlds. Dual control modes can switch between pressure control and volume control during or between breaths. They attempt to deliver a target tidal volume, while regulating the pressure with each breath. To achieve this, the ventilator will make adjustments to the pressure level delivered, based on the compliance and resistance inside the patient's lungs.

PRVC Mode (Similar modes include VC+, Auto flow, and Adaptive Support Ventilation)

Pressure regulated volume control gives the patient full support for both the machine set breaths and the spontaneous breaths, just like A/C mode. What makes PRVC unique is that it adjusts the pressure it uses to reach the set tidal volume. This is pressure regulation and results in lower pressures inside the lung.

When is PRVC used? PRVC is used in patients who require maximum ventilatory support and who need a consistent tidal volume, while using the lowest possible pressures.

Important notes regarding PRVC: Just like A/C mode, PRVC can cause hyperventilation of your patient should they breathe high enough over the set respiratory rate. As noted, PRVC is similar to VC+ on Puritan Bennett ventilators, Auto Flow on Evita XL and Draeger ventilators, and Adaptive Pressure Ventilation on Galileo and Hamilton ventilators.

How does PRVC work? PRVC automatically adjusts itself according to changes in airway resistance and compliance. A specific start-up sequence occurs when PRVC mode is first initiated. The first breath given is a volume-controlled test breath with a pause time set to 10%. During this pause time, the ventilator measures the pressure used to hold in the breath. This pause pressure is then used as the pressure level for the next breath. PRVC is a patient or time-triggered, flow decelerating, pressure or time-cycled mode of ventilation. In addition, PRVC is technically considered a dual control mode. That means both volume and pressure are actively controlled by the ventilator.

Automode

This mode is available on the Maquet Servo-i and Servo 300 ventilators. Auto-mode switches back and forth between a control mode and a spontaneous mode, depending upon the patient's efforts. Starting in a control mode, when the patient triggers two consecutive breaths, Automode switches the patient over to a spontaneous mode. If the patient becomes apneic, the mode is switched back to the original control mode. The control mode can be volume control, PRVC, or pressure control. Volume control and PRVC switch to volume support, while pressure control will switch to pressure support.

When is Automode used?

Automode is used to wean the patient from the ventilator based on the amount of the patient's spontaneous effort. The potential advantage Automode offers is to begin weaning the patient from the ventilator as soon as possible.

Volume Support Mode

This is a spontaneous mode of ventilation in which a target tidal volume is set, and pressure support is auto regulated in proportion to the patient's effort. No respiratory rate is set in volume support ventilation.

How does volume support work? In volume support mode, pressure support will be delivered to the patient at a variable level to achieve a set target tidal volume. When the patient initiates their first breath in volume support mode, that breath will be supported with 10cm H20 pressure. Afterwards, the ventilator continually calculates and adjusts the pressure support by a maximum of 3cm H20 to achieve the target tidal volume. Exhalation starts when the upper pressure limit is exceeded or when the flow decreases below the inspiratory cycle of time. Because both volume and pressure are actively controlled by the ventilator, volume support is a dual control mode of ventilation.

When is volume support used?
Volume support is used to wean patients from mechanical ventilation. Patients in which target volume or minute ventilation is desired may benefit from this mode.

Important notes: Spontaneous modes must be used with caution. Apnea and other alarm limits must be set appropriately to ensure a patient is adequately ventilated. Close observation and monitoring of the patient is always a must while using these modes. In addition, some studies suggest volume support can lead to respiratory distress in patients with an increased ventilatory demand. Therefore, correct selection and monitoring of patients is important when using this mode.

High Frequency Ventilation

The two most common types of high frequency ventilation (HFV) in use today include high frequency oscillatory ventilation and high frequency jet ventilation. Though there are no large controlled randomized studies demonstrating a reduction in morbidity and mortality, the benefits of HFV to specific patient populations have been well documented.

High Frequency Oscillatory Ventilation

High frequency oscillatory ventilation (HFOV) is an unconventional form of ventilation used to reduce or prevent further lung injury in patients with respiratory distress syndrome (IRDS, ARDS). HFOV is commonly

used in neonates. HFOV use in
adults is controversial.

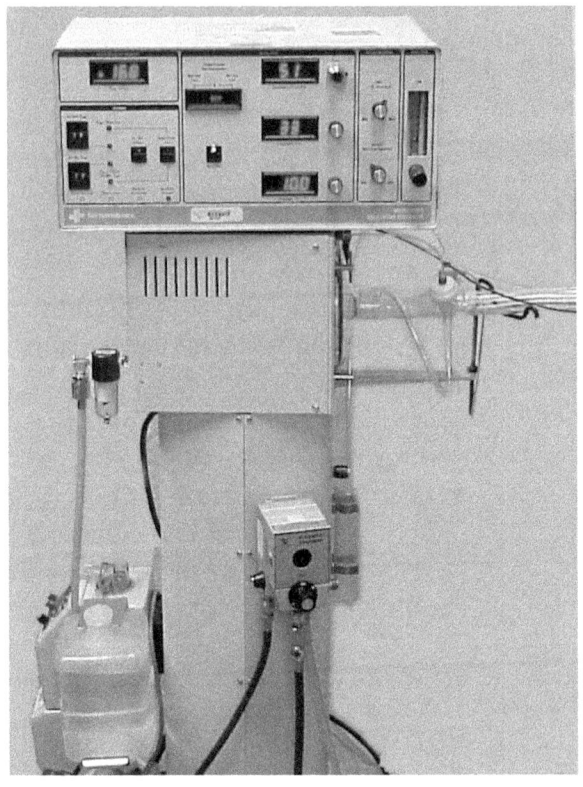

How does HFOV work? - HFOV
uses high respiratory rates,
between 210 and 900 breaths per
minute, with high mean airway
pressure to achieve gentle
ventilation while recruiting alveoli.
The tidal volumes used in HFOV

are extremely small and produced from the oscillations of a diaphragm. Picture how a speaker vibrates when the bass is turned up.

When should I use HFOV? There are no universally accepted indications for high frequency ventilation. However, HFOV is used in neonates and children with IRDS (infant respiratory distress syndrome) and adults with ARDS (acute respiratory distress syndrome). Using HFOV in adults is controversial, as studies have been limited by small sample sizes and poor study design. Ferguson, et al. (2013) published a study in the *New England Journal of Medicine*, which concluded in adults with moderate to severe ARDS, early application of HFOV does not reduce mortality and may increase it. Another study by Young et al. (2013) concluded the use of HFOV had no significant effect on 30-day mortality in patients with acute respiratory distress syndrome (ARDS).

Initial settings

There are at least five protocols in use, regarding the initial settings and ventilation strategies for HFOV. No consensus exists in its initial setup and application. Therefore, initial settings and ventilation strategies are largely determined by clinician familiarity and hospital preference.

Paw (mean airway pressure) - The Paw influences the oxygenation of the patient, much like PEEP.

Amplitude (Delta-P) - This affects the tidal volumes and influences the carbon dioxide.

Hertz (Frequency) - This setting is inverse to the size of the baby. Heavier babies require lower hertz settings. 1 hertz is equal to 60 breaths per minute.

Percent inspiratory time - This is the time the piston is driving forward and ranges between 30 and 50%.

Bias flow - Controls the flow rate of humidified blended gas throughout the ventilator circuit.

FiO2 - The oxygen level is set per hospital protocol.

High Frequency Jet Ventilation

High frequency jet ventilation (HFJV) is an unconventional form of ventilation used to reduce or prevent further lung injury in neonates with respiratory distress syndrome (IRDS, ARDS). HFJV can only be used in the neonatal population.

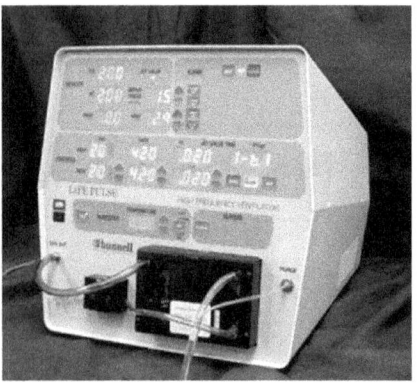

How does Jet ventilation work?

The life pulse HFJV delivers rapid pulses of fresh gas to create tidal volumes of about 1 ml/kg.

Because these tidal volumes are so small, higher levels of PEEP can be used, while preventing over-distension of alveoli. A special ETT adaptor contains a jet port for breath delivery and a pressure monitoring port.

HFJV also allows passive exhalation, which results in enhanced mucociliary clearance of secretions and a lower mean airway pressure as compared to HFOV. The HFJV requires the use of a conventional mechanical ventilator to provide PEEP and sigh breaths.

When should I use Jet ventilation?

HFJV has been used in the neonatal population to treat pulmonary interstitial emphysema (PIE). In neonates with PIE, HFJV has been demonstrated to reduce air leak and help the lung heal as compared to conventional ventilation (Keszler M., et al.).

Initial Jet Settings

The following initial settings guidelines are taken directly from

Bunnells 4-step quick start guide
http://www.bunl.com/quick-start-guide.html. As always, follow a physicians order and/or your hospital protocol.

Jet Rate: Start with 420 bpm. Start lower if patient is larger than 1 kg or is suffering from lung conditions that may cause gas trapping. Selecting rates in multiples of 60 bpm (1 Hz) is convenient.

Jet PIP: Start with PIP equal to or a few cm H2O less than that currently being employed by CMV (or HFOV, as revealed by pre-HFJV monitoring with the Jet in standby mode).

Jet I: Time: Start with default setting of 0.020 sec.

Conventional Ventilator Settings
PEEP: Raise PEEP by 2 cm H2O when transitioning from CMV in order to preserve MAP and lung volume. Adjust PEEP as necessary to maintain same or slightly lower MAP when transitioning from HFOV.

Rate: Start with 5 bpm

PIP: Keep current CMV PIP setting or reduce by 10-50% if concerned about lung injury. If transitioning from HFOV, set CMV PIP a few cm H2O below HFJV PIP.

I: Time: Keep current CMV setting or set at ~ 0.4 sec or less if transitioning from HFOV.

Important notes regarding Jet ventilation:

- Jet ventilators can be used in combination with a nitric oxide delivery system.
- The Jet vent must be placed in standby mode when suctioning or administering surfactant.
- Jet ventilators require the use of a separate conventional ventilator to provide PEEP and sigh breaths.
- Bunnell provides a very impressive interactive feature on its' website. You can practice inputting and adjusting initial settings

here:
http://www.bunl.com/interactive-jet.html

- Bunnell also staffs a hotline for any and all patient care questions relating to the Jet ventilator 24 hours a day at 800-800-4358.

Weaning Modes

CPAP

CPAP stands for Continuous positive airway pressure. CPAP is a simple mode that causes a great deal of confusion because it can be used and applied for entirely different reasons. CPAP can be a weaning mode for intubated patients on mechanical ventilation, or it can be applied with a tight fitting facemask as a treatment for sleep apnea or heart failure. There is no respiratory rate or tidal volume set while using CPAP. In fact, there is no ventilation provided at all by CPAP. Therefore, the patient must be able to spontaneously breathe independently while on this mode.

How does CPAP work? CPAP applies a constant set pressure during both inhalation and exhalation. When CPAP is delivered via an invasive airway, the pressure is transmitted throughout the ventilator circuit, through the patient's airways and eventually to the patient's alveoli. The pressure applied to the alveoli may help recruit collapsed alveoli and maintain alveoli that are patent.

When is CPAP used? CPAP is delivered both invasively and non-invasively, but for very different reasons. CPAP is used invasively as a final step before extubating or disconnecting a patient from the ventilator.

Pressure Support Ventilation

Pressure support, which can be used with CPAP or SIMV, gives the patient extra support for the spontaneous breaths they take. Imagine what it would feel like waking up in a strange hospital bed, unable to talk, your wrists restrained, you're probably in a fair amount of pain or discomfort, and to top it all off, you have to breathe through a long straw. If this ever happens to you, hopefully, you have a great therapist, nurse, or doctor who will recognize your predicament and come to your aid by adding pressure support to your ventilator.

How does PSV work? When the patient triggers a spontaneous breath, a constant pressure is applied to the lungs, causing gas to flow into them. When the flow decreases to a predetermined level, the breath will end and exhalation will begin. This predetermined level is an additional setting, commonly known as the cycle off level.

Breathing through an endotracheal tube causes an increase in airway resistance due to turbulent airflow. PSV helps to overcome that airway resistance by providing a constant pressure to the lungs above the PEEP level. This causes air to flow into the lungs and complements the patient's own efforts to breathe.

When is PSV used, and how do I set it? PSV is used to support a patient's spontaneous breaths in either SIMV mode or CPAP. Pressure support is usually set between 5 and 20 cm H20. The higher the number, the more support is provided. The level of pressure support is often determined by observing the patient's tidal volume. An important concept to remember when using high levels of PSV is that the more PSV the patient requires, the more likely they are not ready for extubation. PSV is not used in A/C mode because all the breaths in A/C mode are completely supported with a set tidal volume.

Non-invasive Modes

BiPAP

Mechanical ventilation can be applied invasively with a variety of airways such as endotracheal, naso-tracheal, or tracheostomy tubes. Mechanical ventilation can also be applied noninvasively using a full face or nasal mask. This non-invasive form of ventilation is achieved through BiPAP or bi-level positive airway pressure.

With BiPAP, a high pressure is applied when the patient inhales, and a lower pressure is applied when they exhale. These two pressures account for the **Bi** part of **Bi**PAP. The greater the difference between inhalation and exhalation pressures, the greater the level of support or ventilation. The PAP portion of Bi**PAP** stands for positive airway pressure.

Though BiPAP is used primarily as a non-invasive means of ventilation, it can also be applied invasively using an advanced airway.

BiPAP is often used to stabilize a patient who is still responsive, able to protect their airway, and suffering from a reversible cause of respiratory failure such as CHF. BiPAP is not intended as a long-term ventilation strategy. BiPAP is often poorly tolerated by patients when used for long-term ventilation, as they will eventually develop BiPAP fatigue.

Skin breakdown around the area the facemask is applied is also common in patients requiring BiPAP greater than 48 hours.

Though non-invasive ventilation has been proven to be effective in preventing intubation of the airway, it has clear contraindications to its use:

- Unresponsive patients who cannot protect their airway

- Apnea or decreased drive to breathe
- Acute sinusitis or otitis media
- Hypotension
- Pneumothorax, Pneumomediastinum
- Epistaxis
- Recent facial, oral or skull surgery/trauma

Extreme caution should be exercised in patients where vomiting is a risk. With the face mask strapped tightly to the patients face, vomiting inside the mask poses a serious risk for aspiration as the vomit becomes trapped inside the mask and becomes forcibly ventilated into the patient's lungs thereafter. Proper humidification of the BiPAP patient's airway is important for patient tolerance. Claustrophobia, which is often exacerbated when patients are short of breath, can often result in a patient's refusal to wear a BiPAP mask.

CPAP

Continuous positive airway pressure can also be applied non-invasively with a nasal or facemask. Non-invasive CPAP is used to treat sleep apnea and heart failure. In patients with heart failure the pressure generated by CPAP helps decrease the work of breathing and decreases pulmonary congestion by moving fluid back into the vascular system. CPAP can treat sleep apnea by using pressure to splint open the patient's airway. Splinting the airway open prevents collapse of the airway and subsequent apnea.

Weaning Parameters

There is no particular weaning parameter or protocol that can predict a successful extubation with 100% accuracy. However, there are numerous measurements and data we can obtain to help ensure a successful extubation. This data is often combined with a physician's clinical judgment and experience to determine if a patient is ready to be extubated.

RSBI - The rapid shallow breathing index is obtained by dividing the patient's total respiratory rate (also known as frequency) by the tidal volume. To calculate the RSBI of a patient with a total respiratory rate of 20 breaths per minute and a tidal volume of 500 ml's, we would divide 20 by .500. The result would be 40. An RSBI below 105 is normal and a good predictor for successful extubation.

However, for RSBI to be accurate, it should be measured as originally intended on a T-piece. A T-piece consists of corrugated tubing, which provides non-pressurized humidified oxygen to the endotracheal or tracheostomy tube. Studies have shown that measuring RSBI on CPAP and/or pressure support can give a false low reading and cause clinicians to extubate patients who are not ready.

NIF (also known as maximum inspiratory pressure or MIP) - Negative inspiratory force reflects the strength of the diaphragm and other muscles of respiration. NIF can be measured through a ventilator by performing an expiratory hold after they have fully exhaled. NIF can also be measured using a handheld manometer. The manometer is connected to the breathing tube, and the greatest negative pressure a patient can generate for at least one second is recorded. Several NIF measurements are attempted, while allowing the patient to rest as needed between measurements. A NIF of at least -20cm H20 is acceptable.

Vital Capacity - VC is measured through the ventilator by instructing the patient at normal end exhalation to take as deep a breath in as possible and then exhale as much of that air as possible. An acceptable VC for extubation is normally considered to be 10-15 ml/kg of ideal body weight, though normal VC values vary, depending on age, sex, height, and ethnicity.

Ventilator Terminology

Volume Control Modes
This is a category of modes that uses a set volume as a target to reach for with each machine-delivered breath.

Pressure Control Modes
This is a category of modes that uses a set pressure to target for with each machine-delivered breath.

Tidal volume
Tidal volume is simply the size of the breath as measured in milliliters. Tidal volume is often calculated based on a patient's ideal body weight. Different lung pathologies will require different sized tidal volumes. Patients with stiff lungs, such as in ARDS, are treated with tidal volumes lower than those with healthy lungs.

Auto-peep

Auto-PEEP is additional pressure remaining in the lungs above the set level of PEEP at the end of exhalation. An expiratory pause maneuver can measure auto-PEEP. Auto-PEEP often results when a patient does not have enough time to fully exhale due to a high set respiratory rate. COPD patients are at high risk of auto-PEEP due to their prolonged expiratory phase.

Auto-Triggering
An auto trigger occurs when a breath is unintentionally given. This is most often due to the flow or pressure trigger being set at too sensitive a level.

Cycling
Cycling refers to what makes the ventilator stop giving the breath. Cycling ends the machine-delivered breath and allows the patient to exhale.

Total Cycle Time
The total cycle time is the time it takes for a patient to inhale and exhale. When the patient begins to receive a breath, the total cycle time begins. When they have

completely exhaled, the total cycle time ends.

I-time

I time stands for inspiratory time. This is the length of time a patient inhales from the beginning of the breath to the moment they stop inhaling. <u>I time can be a very important setting</u>, particularly for your patient's comfort. Imagine being awake on a ventilator. This is a pretty scary thing to begin with. Then, imagine taking a breath in and the ventilator not letting you exhale it when you want to. This can produce a lot of anxiety for your patient, plus it can also cause high peak airway pressures within their lungs if they try to exhale forcefully, before the ventilator is done giving the breath.

E-time

E time stands for expiratory time. This is the length of time it takes for a patient to exhale. The E time is not set directly. The length of the E-time depends on how many breaths you are trying to fit into a minute, and the length of the inspiratory time. The higher the set respiratory rate and/or inspiratory time, the less time a patient has to exhale. This is important in patients with COPD because they already have enough trouble getting air out of their lungs. If they are not given a long enough time to exhale, then they may trap even more air inside their lungs. This can lead to a very uncomfortable COPD ventilator patient, plus negative side effects such as auto-PEEP and high peak airway pressures.

I:E Ratio

This is the ratio of inhalation and exhalation. A normal I:E ratio is 1:3. This means for every 1 second the patient inhales, they are allowed 3 seconds to exhale.

Peak airway pressure (Paw)
Paw is measured and displayed on most ventilators with each breath. Paw reflects the pressure within the patient's large airways and results from is the result of airway resistance and compliance.

Plateau pressure (Pplat)
Plateau pressure measures the pressure applied to the small airways of the lung and alveoli during an inspiratory pause. Plateau pressure reflects how compliant the lungs are. The more compliant the lungs are, the easier they are to inflate. Stiff lungs have poor compliance and are difficult to inflate. When airway resistance increases, a large difference will be seen between the plateau pressures and the peak airway pressures. Many things can cause a large difference between the peak and plateau pressures (for example, bronchospasm and/or secretions in the airways).

Plateau pressure is measured by performing a 0.5 to 1 second inspiratory pause maneuver. To prevent barotrauma, the target plateau pressure is ideally less than 30 cm H20. Things to remember to improve the accuracy of your plateau pressure measurement include making sure the patient is not breath stacking. Make sure the patient has fully exhaled before performing the inspiratory pause maneuver. Also, any leaks within the ventilator circuit or from chest tubes will give an inaccurate result.

Rise Time
This setting determines how fast peak inspiratory flow or pressure is reached during each breath. This can be an important setting for patient comfort.

Airway Resistance (Raw)
This is a measurement of the resistance to air flow throughout the patient's airways. When an asthmatic's bronchial tubes constrict, the airway resistance to flow increases. When the asthma patient is given a bronchodilator, their airway resistance decreases as the airways dilate or widen.

Secretions in the airways also increase airway resistance. The speed you deliver the breath can also increase airway resistance. For example, a high flow rate causes more turbulent airflow. Turbulent airflow increases the airway resistance. A lower flow rate creates laminar flow, which moves through the airways with ease as compared to turbulent airflow.

Compliance

Compliance refers to the lungs' ease of distension. High compliance means a lung can be easily inflated. Low compliance means a lung is stiff and hard to inflate.

Flow rate

The peak flow rate is the maximum amount of gas that can flow through the ventilator circuit during inspiration. This value is normally expressed in Liters per minute.

More By The Author

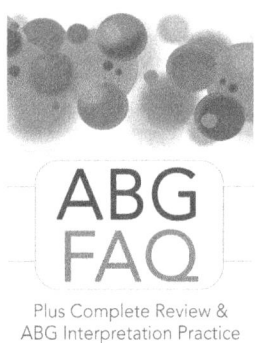

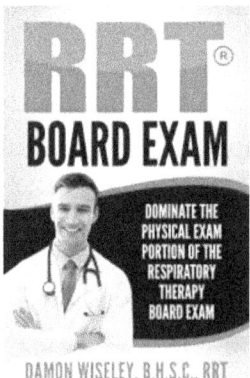

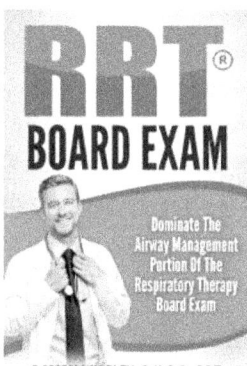

RRT®

BOARD EXAM

Dominate The
Airway Management
Portion Of The
Respiratory Therapy
Board Exam

DAMON WISELEY, B.H.S.C., RRT

RRT®

BOARD EXAM

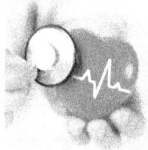

Dominate The
Cardiac Portion
of the RRT
Board Exams

DAMON WISELEY, B.H.S.C., RRT

For more FREE tips, tricks, and courses designed to help you gain confidence with respiratory therapy topics, please visit our main website @

www.rtboardexam.com

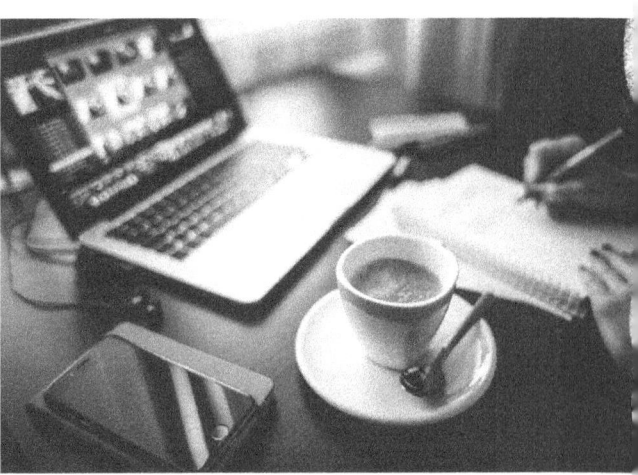

References

Ferguson, N. D., Cook, D. J., Gordon, H. G., Sangeeta M. S., Hand, L., Austin, P., Meade, M. O. (2013). High Frequency Oscillation in Early Acute Respiratory Distress Syndrome. *The New England Journal of Medicine*, 368(9), 795-805. doi: 10.1056/NEJmoa1215554

Young, D., Lamb, S. E., Shah, S., MacKenzie, L., Tunnicliffe, M., Ranjit, L., Rowan, K., Cuthbertson, B. H. (2013). High-Frequency Oscillation for Acute Respiratory Distress Syndrome. *The New England Journal of Medicine*, 368,(9) 806-813. doi: 10.1056/NEJMoa1215716

Keszler M, Donn SM, Bucciarelli RLL, et al. A multicentered trial comparing high-frequency jet ventilation and conventional mechanical ventilation in newborn infants with pulmonary interstitial emphysema. J Pediatr. 1991;119:85-93.